Brainb...

Left-handedness
and
Growing up with
Neurodevelopmental
Delay

Sue Cook

DEDICATION

I dedicate this book to my parents who have been the
inspiration for this book in different ways.
I dedicate this book to Svea Gold.
I dedicate this book to India Robins.
I dedicate this book to the lefthanders of this world.
I dedicate this book to the idea that the individual can
make a difference.
And to my children.
And to Rob Ryan.

CONTENTS

ACKNOWLEDGMENTS

Thank you to my proof readers, my Dad and my stepfather Keith Redfern.

Thank you to my family for believing in me.
Thank you to my friends, you have supported me, even though you might not be aware of that.

Thank you to Caroline Anthony for being the first person to buy my first book, and giving me a five star rating on Amazon. Thank you for encouraging me to do more books.

Thank you Rob Ryan for the continued support and calmness. You are a joy.

1 LEFTHANDERS

Lefthandedness only affects about ten per cent of the population directly but it actually affects more than that. If there is a leftie in a family, then the whole family needs to be aware of what life is like for that person.

Or if you have a child who is a leftie, you need to understand them better too. I do know how it feels to have a child with learning difficulties, and I do know what it is like to help them. I hope you find the following interesting....

Left handers are not wrong. We are just different. Accept it. In my family, growing up, there were two lefties and two righties. My mother and I are the left handers. It was a democratic household.

We had left handed scissors and right handed scissors. Nobody was teased for being the odd one out. Our differences were appreciated and discussed, not mocked. I have been laughed at by righties, and called Cack handed. Cack is not a pleasant insult. And all because the brain is wired differently.

Odd isn't it? That is not acceptable to me, that people are verbally abused because of what boils down to ignorance.

I am probably one of the lucky ones, having grown up in a democratically handed household. But for many children, they are misunderstood, blamed, insulted, and not catered for. And that is ten per cent of the population.

If I say to you now 'lefthanders are different and have different needs' how do you react? If you are a right hander you might be thinking that this is nonsense and a stupid comment. But imagine being on the receiving end of that negativity when you do have genuinely different needs....

When my friends find out that I have left handed cooking equipment and left handed knives, and scissors, and rulers, they laugh. It is a total mystery that anyone should need such bizarre things.

But they have them automatically as a right hander, and do not even realise it. Everything we buy has been designed by someone, and where relevant, it is designed to be used by a right hander. So therefore it penalises the lefty. Accidentally.

I'm really hoping the Science Museum does a left hander room one day so the righties can try everything out and see for themselves what life through the looking glass is like. Cartons of milk are right handed (try pouring them with your left hand and you will see what I mean).

I have a left handed corkscrew and all the right handers cut themselves on it, so I have stopped using it. My friends cut themselves on my knives too, even when I warn them, they still cut themselves.

This is not meant to be a moan, rather an explanation of the hidden difficulties we have. Injuries and insults as well as awkwardness.

When I was at university I wrote a literature review on handedness and intelligence. I wanted to know if we really were stupid as lefthanders as we were so often told. I found out that we are not, we are often more intelligent than righties, except if we have brain damage.

So, aside from the scissors and knives, and injury potential, I like being lefthanded. So do my leftie friends.

We make the best of it. We feel it gives us an edge; we think differently, we come to different conclusions, we are far from ordinary. And I will explain why.

2 HOW LEFTHANDERS LEARN

Left handers differ from right handers more than just by writing with the other hand.

There are two hemispheres, or sides, in the brain. Right handers have a left hemisphere that is dominant, in most cases, and left handers have a dominant right hemisphere in most cases.

Each hemisphere does slightly different things from the other, like non identical twins perhaps. So that means that left handers do not think in the same way as right handers, and they most certainly learn differently.

School is designed to teach right handers, after all they are around 90% of the population.

Right handers learn by looking at detail and then more detail and building it up into a picture. I often describe this to people as 'mosaic learning'. Each piece builds the picture. Sound familiar?

Left handers learn by looking at the whole picture,

seeing the scope of the subject, and then by looking at detail. We need to see the whole mosaic and then look at the individual pieces.

So, in a classroom where the detail is presented first, left handers are constantly searching for the whole picture to make sense of the subject, and it is not until the end of the term that they can see the whole picture and suddenly things make sense, if they are lucky.

So left handers are at a disadvantage at school.

If your child is left handed and you want to help them, what can you do? Ensure that they have the correct equipment. Left handed writing implements can be very helpful. Other useful tools are rulers and scissors.

Also, tell them the whole picture first and the details last. This is hard for right handers to do. But it will give you an insight into how hard things are for us.

3 WHAT THE HEMISPHERES DO
Usual hemispheric localisation of function

Left handers gestalt function	Right handers
right cerebral hemisphere	left cerebral hemisphere
visual recognition of faces, shapes, colour, objects, pictographs	word recognition
space, shape, direction (visuospatial)	understanding- concepts
drawing musical appreciation intonational pattern imposed on speech; singing	Reading writing Spelling arithmetic, number
constructional praxis	speech
facial expression gesture recognition manipulative and spatial (visuomotor)	verbal reasoning
flight	fight

Very young children have not yet become well lateralised. If we were forced to learn with a brain that had matching hemispheres until we went to school (rather than a brain that had different skills on each side), speaking, reading, writing, and drawing would be prevented from developing

properly.
Here are a few examples of the problems that would show.

Reversal when copying shapes.
Reversal of patterns
Right/left confusion
Difficulty with imitation of gestures
Speech reversals in words, sound or phrase
Reading reversal: saw/was god/dog
Writing reversal; b/d on/no
Suppression of one eye with squint
(Kingsley Whitmore 1999)

So in other words, we NEED the two sides to do different things, or we would be stuck in a frustrating world with a stunted mind.
You can see from the list above that these are symptoms often found in children with learning difficulties as they often do not have a dominant hemisphere yet.

'The question of dominance has been debated for years. Just recently the OEP, Optometric Extension Service, did a big study. They found that reading was not affected by whether a person was totally right or totally left, but in those with mixed dominance there were more problems with reading. Using the opposite eye from the hand, if nothing else gives you a kink in the neck. Also it is hard when you try to hammer something and don't know with which hand to pick up the hammer.

'Mixed dominance means something was wrong in the earlier development.' Quote from Svea Gold in her correspondence to me in 2007.
But if your child IS differentiated, and is left handed...
The first step in helping your left handed child, is

therefore to ACCEPT.
ACCEPT them for who and what they are. ACCEPT
them for their difference.
And
ALLOW your child to BE THEMSELVES.
ALLOW yourself to appreciate their differences; they
are not like you.

In the course of my studies on handedness I have
read dozens of books and read hundreds of scientific
peer reviewed research articles in science
magazines. Some of these books gave a gloomy
picture of left handedness. But they were written by
right handers. How can they know what it is like?
They can't. But, statistically, left handers do have
more accidents, more allergies, wear glasses and die
a bit younger. This is due to living in a world
designed to trip us up constantly. Researchers are
not sure why lefties have more allergies though.

Having a dominant hemisphere is very important if
the brain is to be able to mature and grow and
'specialise'. Otherwise it is stuck in a more primitive
state.

This is very awkward, and results in the confusions
and reversals known in dyslexic states. So there can
be only one boss in the brain; a dominant
hemisphere. Otherwise there is chaos (it is like a car
having two drivers).

The exercises in the programme I teach give the
brain a chance to develop a dominant side. One
sided sports such as tennis or bowling help the brain
to specialise.

Usually if a person is left handed they are right
hemisphere dominant and vice versa but not always.

Occasionally there is a person with a dominant hemisphere and same side dominant hand, when there is strong dominance in the person and not mixed dominance.

My father and my son are two examples. These two do not fit any of the usual categories mentioned and are unusual thinkers. For more information read Carla Hannaford's book The Dominance Factor).
http://handedness.org/action/leftwrite.html

4 The Hemispheres

It is important that we use both hemispheres, not just one, but IN AN ORGANISED WAY. If there is no hemispheric dominance there is poor organisation of the neural pathways, and poor development too. This will result in chaos. So the aim is to improve this so that the brain can function in its most optimum way using both hemispheres. It is important to say that to clear up any confusion.

Here is what Svea Gold had to say on the subject in 2007 *'The neurologist Norman Geschwind had a lot to say about handedness. Life is so much easier when you know with what hand to pick up a hammer. The difficulty in establishing dominance is that you are never quite sure whether this child was meant to be right or left at birth. Lyelle Palmer says that we teach a child to be right handed but don't teach foot dominance, so that is a clue. However, if the child has not established dominance by age six it is a sign that something in the lower development of the brain is not organized properly, and once you fix that, the child may change handedness on his own. Now that we no longer force a left handed child to be right, we no longer see the huge amount of stuttering we did when I was young.*
I used to think that if a child was fully one sided - ah, that's great I don't have to worry about that, but

then I found that sometimes they do not use the other side at all! Anyhow, don't try to learn it all at once - it takes a couple of hundred years. Just remember that no two kids are alike, but the normal developmental progression always remains the same.
Svea'

One annoying thing that I do as a left hander in a right handed world, is when I am at the front of a queue, I turn away to the left and bump in to the person standing behind me who is expecting me to turn to the right like everybody else. Then I end up in a mix of people instead of in a clear path out.

In 2008 research (Battles, 2008) economists at University College Dublin found that left handed men were earning 4% per hour more than the right handers. This is attributed to our ability to adapt, claims the secretary of the Left Handers Club of Ireland. Left handed women though, were earning 4% less than the right handers. It looks like adaptation is something men are able to benefit from in the workplace, whereas women are not.

Scientist Chris McManus, (Griffiths August 2003 Sunday Times Online) says that schools are still failing left handers by ignoring the fact that they are different, but in the past children were punished for it. He says 15 to 20% of left handers are dyslexic. And he says that it might be desirable to fast track gifted left handers.

And yet 'southpaw scholarships' are available. There are many scholarships accessible specifically for left-handed scholars when you look carefully. A Frederick and Mary F. Beckley Scholarship for up to a thousand dollars is available at Juniata College in Huntington,

Pennsylvania. Awarded to students attending Juniata College and it was established in the seventies, this college scholarship has aided over forty left-handed students through school.

Other differences in the way we think include this piece of news from June 2009, *'A recent study in Neuropsychology shows that the brains in left handed people make connections between their left and right hemispheres quicker. This faster movement allows left handers to deal with situations where they are faced with multiple tasks, such as gaming, more efficiently.'*

Researchers from the Australian National University obtained this information by measuring the transfer time between the two sides of the brain. Test subjects carried out tasks that required them to use both sides of their brains, and it emerged that left handers reacted up to 43 milliseconds faster than right handers.

I agree with this, I can think really quickly sometimes, much faster than most people. I always found this very handy in exams; I never failed to finish on time. But when numbers or certain processing are involved my whole system crashes (I am dyscalculate).

A recent piece of research found that left handed surgeons (residents) were *'more likely to perform eye surgery without complications'*. Surgical resident's dominant hand may influence outcomes of cataract extraction.

J Cataract Refract Surg. 2009;35(6):1019-1025

The Anything Left handed website has an interesting survey with results, and also a 'How Lefthanded are you? test to do with your right handed friends.

At the Handedness Research Institute MK Holder PhD has written an article called Teaching Left-Handers to Write. He states it is not the opposite of teaching a right hander, that it is more difficult to write with the left hand. There are good instructions to help. http://handedness.org/action/leftwrite.html

I am a lefthander. I am also left eared and this is a problem due the organisation of the brain. Lefthanders are not just a mirror image of right handers. I have explained the problems with left earedness below.

5 LATERALITY ISSUES

A right eared person will hear something and the sound information will (in most cases) pass straight into the left hemisphere where it is decoded. A left eared person will hear something and the sound travels into the right hemisphere and then back into the left hemisphere. The result can be 'auditory delay'. Someone might say to me 'are you going to the cinema tonight?' and I will hear 'are you going … ……….ight'.

I miss what always seems like the important bit of the sentence. Even when it is repeated several times I always miss the same bit. So the question is, do I try to change my earedness and mess up my hemispheric dominance? So I answer the phone with my right ear and I don't miss bits.

It didn't surprise me when this piece of research was published 'Researchers at University "Gabriele d'Annunzio" in Chieti, Italy have published the results of three cleverly designed studies that indicate that humans are more apt to act on information heard through their right ears than through their left'. Probably, this is due to the auditory delay I mentioned and the message getting lost.

In the following piece of research, brain wiring with regard to laterality is discussed. But for a more in depth look at this, see Carla Hannaford's Right Moves, and also, The Dominance Factor.
http://www.register-herald.com/local/local_story_067212856.html
Fred Pace

Another problem that seems to happen in left handers with neurodevelopment issues is problems with maths. I have written an article entitled Being Dyscalculate which is in a separate book (brainbuzzz:the evolution).

Being dyscalculate is a nuisance. My school teachers shouted at me because they couldn't believe I didn't understand what they were trying to teach. Why can't an otherwise bright girl do such a simple thing?

Being left handed doesn't help either because our eyes naturally scan from right to left. With words it is OK because the brain knows them so well, there is familiarity, though occasionally I have transposed parts of a word. For years I thought vitamin B6 was called Pyroxidine, not pyridoxine.

But with numbers, there is no consistency, they can be anything, so I usually transpose them or just get them in the wrong order.

Numbers are a total mystery. I am told there are patterns to numbers and that they are logical. Numbers to me are like a foreign language that I have never been able to translate. I cannot decode it.

It is very important when dealing with children with

these problems that we accept them for who they are. They do not choose these problems but are forced to live with them. We as parents can facilitate their growth with patience, understanding, acceptance and love.

I know how hard it is. I have learning difficulties and am a parent of someone who had them too.

This is why I am SO driven to help others. THERE ARE ANSWERS. The Brainbuzzz programme provides you with what you need.

Sally Goddard Blythe (2009) explains dyscalculia as being a situation where '*a solution to a mathematical problem requires both hemispheres to work together. Carrying out a simple arithmetic calculation can involve up to nine changes in hemispheric dominance, together with the ability to sequence (cerebellum), to hold number facts in working memory, and to articulate answers using verbal language*'.

That explains why I can be working something out and then the mind is suddenly blank. Nine changes of hemisphere is quite a lot of processing in itself.

References
Jan Battles Left-handed people are 'high earners' Sunday Times online 25 September 2008.

Sian Griffiths Education: The gifted children dealt a poor hand Sunday Times Online August 3 2003.

Clark, Margaret M. 1959. Teaching left-handed children. (NY: Philosophical Library, Inc.)

Cole, Luella. 1955. Handwriting for left-handed

children. (Bloomington, IL: Public School Publishing Co.)

Gardner, Warren H. 1945. Left handed writing instruction manual. (Danville, IL: The Interstate).

Szeligo, F., B. Brazier, and J. Houston. 2003. Adaptations of writing posture in response to task demands for left- and right-handers. Laterality, 8(3): 261-276.

Holder, M.K. (2003). Teaching left-handers how to write. Handedness Research Institute papers. URL: handedness.org/action/leftwrite.html

Kingsley Whitmore, Hilary Hart, Guy Willems (1999) A Neurodevelopmental Approach to Specific Learning Disorders Cambridge University Press.

Goddard Blythe S. (2009) Attention Balance and Coordination. Wiley Blackwell

http://www.register-herald.com/local/local_story_067212856.html
Fred Pace
Resources
Anything Left handed
PO Box 46
Witney
OX29 7HD
UK
www.anythingleft-handed.co.uk
0845 8723272

http://www.neurodiversity.com/lefthandedness.html

PART TWO

GROWING UP WITH NEURODEVELOPMENTAL DELAY

6 MY FATHER'S STORY

What happens if you don't treat adhd and dyslexia and other problems like this? It is possible to live a normal life with brain wiring problems? My father is a great example of this as you will find out here. This is his story. He has ADHD and has never had it treated. So I have included it here because it is such a great inspiration and hope to parents everywhere.

I think it is a bit like going through life with a faulty gear box to not have any treatment. Supposing second gear never worked; driving would not be as fluent or as safe as it could be, and it could cause accidents. Or supposing second and third never worked? It would be extremely awkward. But that is what it is like for these children, awkward, difficult and sometimes dangerous.

The brain rewiring exercises would be like making the gears smooth; you can use the whole engine without sudden problems....Suddenly life can run smoothly.

My father is a great example of this. He was born in 1932. He is deaf, also, and he attributes this mostly to industrial circumstances. He lived in many countries installing diesel engines the size of a small house and often he slept in the engine rooms and had to put up with the noise they made. Diesel engines are very noisy. He also has tinnitus which is a constant ringing and rushing noise in his ears.

As a child his father would say to him 'swing your arms when you walk'. I now know that this means his brain was badly organised and that he had missed some important steps in his neural development.

His teachers caned him because he could not do maths, and they bashed his ears with their hands. This violence is unacceptable and though it does not occur in schools today, the system is still often failing children with reading problems.

Dad is unable to conceptualise history, or time and, cannot arrive anything but half an hour early for any appointment. He does not have any idea about the difference in time between the Victorians and the Stone Age. He can't work it out.

He is a great example for us of someone who is untreated with neurodevelopmental problems, in particular ADHD, and also I hope, an inspiration.

Part of his education occurred during World War Two and as a consequence he was evacuated to Yorkshire from Essex and hardly seemed to go to school.

He left school at 14 without any qualifications and started a seven year engineering apprenticeship.

Compressing the next few years, he did two years National Service as an engineer, then some time later ended up at Marconi in Chelmsford and was soon posted to Angola to install diesel engines, to provide power for microwave radio systems and give towns power for the first time.

In Dad's words *'My work - I mainly installed power*

stations for Microwave radio networks (where I slept in the engine rooms next to the running diesels) and only occasionally helped out with a major power station. But in Canada I built and installed switchgear for major generating stations'.

 Angola, then Ecuador, Angola again and Nigeria (where he met my mother and had my sister), then Venezuela. I came along in Venezuela. Then Newfoundland and Nova Scotia.

After a few years in the UK, he worked in Saudi, and then home again. The reason I have mentioned this is because, in a world where our prisons are full of people with neurodevelopmental problems, here we have a man with no qualifications (at this point) except an apprenticeship, travelling the world, earning money and having staff work for him.

Dad always says he was lucky, it was the sixties, and there was opportunity. But he had a strong work ethic 'you only get out what you put in' and 'be in the right place at the right time' (which he always managed to do).

It was while working in England in the 1970s as a teacher when he discovered the food allergy and intolerance information from the Hyperactive Children Support Group (HACSG). So he was in a good position to help others.

We all knew none of us in our family could do maths, but it wasn't until years after he had trained as a dyslexia teacher that we heard the word dyscalculia. I realised I had it too (and that's another story).

So, looking at Dad objectively and the factors that have compromised his life, and it is the deafness, the maths, ADHD, no sense of history, that have played a big part. Until he was 72 he was working seven days a week teaching dyslexia pupils. He also did voluntary work at Wayland Prison in Norfolk teaching some of the dyslexic inmates.

So he has neurodevelopmental delay that has gone untreated. Also it seems, he is right handed with a dominant right hemisphere (a left hander brain), see Carla Hannaford's The Dominance Factor.

What kept him not only out of prison but the most honest and law abiding person ever (given that our prisons are full of learning disabled people)? Probably opportunity and his skills combined and the fact that he could read very well. He is very competent and a hard worker.

Having neurodevelopmental problems is nothing to do with intelligence, it just affects our ability to use our intelligence in a way that other people take for granted.

Aside from his career, Dad was an inventor, and this is a great example of someone who thinks outside the box. In his case it is more a case of 'what box?'

Dad invented the intermittent windscreen wiper when he was a teenager, but never patented it. He has invented various other useful equipment based items and improved the design on various tools (he is an engineer) but he has never followed these inventions up because he didn't know how. Such a shame.

7 MY EARLY DAYS

There are parallels with my own life here. I was born in 1965 and spent the first two years of my life in Venezuela and the next three in Newfoundland and then Nova Scotia.

Mum was very proud of the fact that I walked at nine months, and she put me in a babywalker when I should have been crawling. Thus my learning problems.

Svea had this to say in 2007 about not crawling '*When you walked too early, the cerebellum was not stimulated. The cells in the cerebellum fire when the target moves at the same time as the head moves... We are treating a brain, not treating the symptom.*'

My school life began in England in 1970. I remember those first few days at school when we did maths.

I remember looking at the blackboard while the teacher pointed to a number with a symbol near another number (a sum such as 2+3=) and was not surprised when people knew the answer. It was a total mystery to me.

No one had told me that numbers had a value (I Just knew them by their names), no one explained the symbol (a plus sign). I realised I was being shown a code but I could not work it out. That is what being dyscalculate is. Non dyscalculate people just know this without having to be told.

I was slow at reading. Mum would not allow phonetics, and as a left hander, I was likely to be slower to master it anyway.

I didn't get to grips with it until I was eight. But once I cracked it, it was like lighting the blue touch paper. I have never stopped reading. I was a magazine editor for much of my twenties which shows that a slow start does not predict the future. When I was eight my top two adult teeth grew out, and that is considered to be the time when reading moves into the right hemipshere and becomes iconic/image based. This observation of teeth growth and reading can be found in an out of print book 'Is my Child in the Wrong Grade?' by Dr Ames. Many children gain their front two teeth at about 7, and that signifies when the brain is properly ready to read.

My year 5 teacher went through a spell of keeping me in at lunchtime to go over the maths with me and she would shout and scream at me. She was so cross that I couldn't understand. I was so terrorised about numbers after this that the mere mention of maths would have me shaking.

And so it stayed like that. I failed maths O level three times, and never achieved a pass. But I tried. Shouting at children is not a teaching method I recommend.

Not being able to do maths has been a dreadful handicap and I had to arrange my life to avoid number interaction.

Part of my hunger to help people overcome their problems is because I can't bear to think of anyone struggling with these things when I know how to help them. The impact of neurodevelopmental delay can be devastating for whole families even if just one member is affected. But our whole family was affected. I didn't know anything else.

Survival instincts are strong in me and I wanted to succeed. I always believed in myself and knew that I was a bright person. One day I would prove it. People are very dismissive of people with learning problems. So I covered up my maths secret and never told anyone. It did get me into trouble occasionally as my judgement with numbers was so off. I made a hugely inaccurate estimate of the cost of something at work once and got told off. They thought I was trying to take advantage, but I was not. Having a problem like this can affect my confidence sometimes. I don't stand up for myself when people criticise me. In other ways I am a very confident person.

Why is this relevant? Because if you are the parent of a child with learning problems you have probably felt despair and hopelessness. For my generation and that of my father, we have slipped through the net, gone undetected and unhelped and we have made our own way through, without being able to do maths and without support. It wasn't easy and we didn't know why it was so hard for us. I sometimes felt like everyone else had an instruction book which made things easy for them. These weren't things I could guess, and some things remained a mystery.

The point of telling you this is to help you not feel despair when your child struggles and you feel like they are not performing to what you expect of them academically. Far too many of our young end up in prison when they have learning difficulties, but there are other journeys they could take, and with or without a neurodevelopment programme like mine, it's not all doom and gloom, as my father's story shows. That said, given the options, I would have preferred not to endure the years of torture I experienced at school. My self esteem was very badly damaged. I'm not sure having parents on the spectrum helped me either as they didn't know how to help.

I realised that balancing 'playing to our strengths' while sorting out the weaknesses, helps a lot. Learn from my mistakes and experience, please, let me teach you neurodevelopment.

8 SENSORY ISSUES

My observation from treating over a hundred children with the neurodevelopment programme I use, is that neurotypical development, is typical in everyone. That may sound obvious, but it needs pointing out. That is why repeating the neurotypical stages in the neurodiverse, results in a brain that is able to function better but does not take anything away from the person.

Sometimes people ask me if doing the programme will take anything away from their child because they have unique gifts. I feel that this needs explaining. There are a lot of wonderful, different, really clever, gifted people with neurodevelopment/spectrum problems. Yes they are talented and amazing individuals. No one would want to change that. I fully acknowledge, praise, support and rejoice in that.

Symptoms of spectrum disorders can be uncomfortable. For example if your pupils are not contracting, they are remaining large, then it is a problem in the brainstem which is where pupillary control comes from. The effect of having large pupils is like snow-blindness. There is far too much light entering the eyes, and it is painful, dazzling, and probably riddled with after images. How can you look anyone in the eye, or focus on anything with snow-blindness? That is an autistic symptom and one that I can show you how to sort out in a few weeks. Gaining pupillary control will have a profound effect on your life because you will now be able to see things. Imagine you are a six year old child and you are painting a picture. Your pupils are massive and your eyes hurt. If you are smart, what do you do? You paint the page black because it eases the snow-blindness. That is a very different conclusion from other ones you may have heard about children painting the page black. That is taking nothing away from a person, but giving a more comfortable life.

Tracking issues, when your eyes cannot follow a moving object while your head is still, will affect your ability to catch a ball, copy from the board, read a line of text, and add up a stack of numbers. Those are academic results of not being able to track, but the social impact is just as great. Children with tracking issues are sometimes clingy at parties, hanging on to their parent, are upset at parties, unable to join in, and generally very unhappy in those situations.

I can show you how to help your child with their tracking and in most cases there is a massive improvement within a month. My son gained tracking skills in a few days and it was life changing because he was able to integrate in social environments for the first time, and to be able to start performing classroom tasks.

My son also had no three dimensional vision. His eyes were not 'yoked' and working as a team. The result was no depth perception. So he had no idea what 'distance' was. He couldn't catch a ball, or feel comfortable in social situations. He gained three dimensional vision in a few weeks of doing the programme.

Vision problems play a massive role in spectrum disorders. And I feel that understanding the impact of these issues, will help you understand that you are taking nothing away from a person by improving their brain organisation.

Our eyes give us so much sensory information and if there is any problem it can have a colossal impact on our lives.

The programme I do with individuals, and teach to groups, works on the entire sensory input to the brain (vision, balance, touch, proprioception, and the rest). It is a sensory programme. When you have dyslexia, dyspraxia, dyscalculia, ADHD, Asperger's, mutism, Autism, you have sensory issues. You have problems with the nerve inputs to the brain.

If the input is problematic, the output will be problematic. So I show you how to correct the input. Simple. We just repeat the neurodevelopmental stages that a neurotypical person automatically does. All that wonderful giftedness that was compromised in a world of pain and limitation, can be released. To me that is a joyful thing, not a negative.

ABOUT THE AUTHOR

Sue Cook is mother to two boys, and lives in Essex. Sue is someone who researches until she finds what she needs, and this collection of books are evidence of that.
Sue learned neurodevelopment to help her son, and then it developed into an accidental practice as her phone began ringing and she refused to turn anyone away who came for help. Thus she has amassed a vast amount of experience and knowledge on this journey and here she shares some of that experience that helped shape her work.

This is the fourth book in the Brainbuzzz series.
The others are:
Brainbuzzz: the evolution;
Nutrition for Special Needs Volumes 1 and 2.
Sue has also published some short stories including: A Gift for Santa and The Good Goblin.